# Still Life

# Still Life

## A Parent's Memoir of Life
## After Stillbirth and Miscarriage

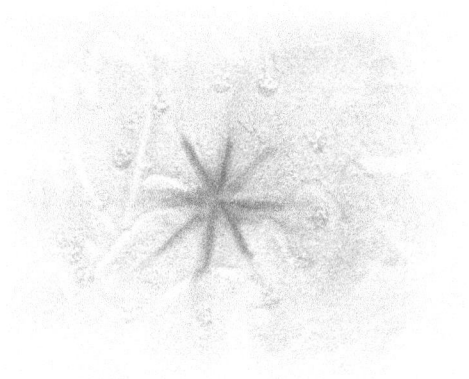

Emma Mellon, PhD

SUNSTONE
PRESS

SANTA FE

Sunstone books may be purchased for educational, business, or sales promotional use.
For information please write: Special Markets Department, Sunstone Press,
P.O. Box 2321, Santa Fe, New Mexico 87504-2321.

Cover art by Damini Celebre

Book design › Vicki Ahl
Body typeface › Constantia
Printed on acid-free paper
∞
eBook 978-1-61139-473-3

---

Library of Congress Cataloging-in-Publication Data

Names: Mellon, Emma, author.
Title: Still life : a parent's memoir of life after stillbirth and
    miscarriage / by Emma Mellon, PhD.
Description: Santa Fe : Sunstone Press, [2016]
Identifiers: LCCN 2016013918 (print) | LCCN 2016022674 (ebook) | ISBN
    9781632931344 (softcover : alk. paper) | ISBN 9781611394733 ()
Subjects: LCSH: Mellon, Emma. | Stillbirth--Psychological aspects. |
    Miscarriage--Psychological aspects. | Parents--Psychology. | Loss
    (Psychology)
Classification: LCC RG648 .M45 2016 (print) | LCC RG648 (ebook) | DDC
    362.198/3920092 [B] --dc23
LC record available at https://lccn.loc.gov/2016013918

---

SUNSTONE PRESS IS COMMITTED TO MINIMIZING OUR ENVIRONMENTAL IMPACT ON THE PLANET.
THE PAPER USED IN THIS BOOK IS FROM RESPONSIBLY MANAGED FORESTS. OUR PRINTER HAS RECEIVED CHAIN OF CUSTODY (COC)
CERTIFICATION FROM: THE FOREST STEWARDSHIP COUNCIL™ (FSC®), PROGRAMME FOR THE ENDORSEMENT OF FOREST CERTIFICATION™
(PEFC™), AND THE SUSTAINABLE FORESTRY INITIATIVE® (SFI®).
THE FSC® COUNCIL IS A NON-PROFIT ORGANIZATION, PROMOTING THE ENVIRONMENTALLY APPROPRIATE, SOCIALLY BENEFICIAL AND
ECONOMICALLY VIABLE MANAGEMENT OF THE WORLD'S FORESTS. FSC® CERTIFICATION IS RECOGNIZED INTERNATIONALLY
AS A RIGOROUS ENVIRONMENTAL AND SOCIAL STANDARD FOR RESPONSIBLE FOREST MANAGEMENT.

---

WWW.SUNSTONEPRESS.COM
SUNSTONE PRESS / POST OFFICE BOX 2321 / SANTA FE, NM 87504-2321 /USA
(505) 988-4418 / ORDERS ONLY (800) 243-5644 / FAX (505) 988-1025

This book is dedicated to
the memory of Janis Keyser,
Executive Director of UNITE.

# Contents

*Koan*

*Stillborn boy drops into the world*

    *like Icarus into the sea,*
    *like a seed into earth,*
    *like a koan into the mind.*

    E.M.

# Foreword

Just as the light of a new star continues through the universe long after its explosive beginning, stillbirth travels through the years of parents' lives. Far beyond pain and grief, the story continues.

Publicly, parents tell the story in concrete and linear details: Now this baby would be five or twenty-five. Today is the anniversary. He is buried in Philadelphia. I always cry when I think of her. I never hear his name spoken. I hung his baby picture with the other children's. We divorced after she died. We established a charity in her name. I still don't drive by that hospital. I keep his little blue blanket in a drawer. I expect my ashes to be combined with his someday.

The deeper story of a stillbirth continues in more private, idiosyncratic experiences not usually talked about because they seem too odd, too personal, too full of meaning or emotion, and too incredible. This inside story is where meaning is made, healing continues, and the ongoing connection with the lost child enriches life.

This book offers the long view of life after stillbirth. The reader joins me in the upheaval and confusion of it and witnesses the new life that emerges. The power of the relationship with my son, before and after death, reorders life, resolves old struggles, burns away distortions, and reveals deep and durable bonds. In *Still Life*, loss and chaos move toward connection and coherence.

My son, Zachary David, died in utero on November 21, 1988, and was born the next day. That I have survived and thrived since his death is still a surprise to me. I can take credit for very little of this new life. I've had to conclude that we are built—physically, emotionally, and spiritually—to experience, to be changed, and to go on to experience more. I am learning that this innate resiliency is part of a larger resilience—a larger, universal life—that holds and nourishes us all.

I hope my story will encourage other bereaved parents to recognize their own inside stories, find their ongoing connections with their children, and be comforted and created anew by them.

# 1

## Stranger in the House

February 2014

First, I felt everything with him. There was nothing that was not him. Then, he was gone. I mourned. Time passed, and I moved on, altered.

Now a different life than I had dreamed of in those days nourishes me.

Here, in my mid-sixties, I thrive. I have a career as a psychologist in private practice that I treasure. My writing gives me deep satisfaction. My family of friends shares the joys and frustrations of my life. And I've been blessed with good health.

And he is as he was: sketched from Polaroid pictures taken at the hospital. The face of an infant, eyes closed, silent and still.

I pass him many times a day. His is the last picture in a series of family photos that climb the wall of the stairway. At the bottom, my grandparents, and then my parents, me as a baby, my favorite aunt and me, and at the top step, my son. As I pass the relatives, and, depending on the day and my mood, I usually feel something—warmth or curiosity or happiness or regret.

For a long time, I have not felt anything when I pass Zachary. He has become a stranger. His image could be the death mask of a child pharaoh, or the face of a sleeping baby in a baroque painting, or an anonymous little boy in those stock photos that come with picture frames. I've wondered if it was time to put the picture away, like you'd do with the photo of an old lover. Why keep it around? That relationship is over.

But that doesn't seem right. He was my son—is my son—even though he's dead. After twenty-six years, can I find him again?

In these stories and reflections, I'll circle back to our beginnings and visit moments between then and now when I've caught glimpses of him and of us. I want to gather up the moments when having had him and lost him nudged me ahead in new directions. I want to understand how is he present in my life now.

# 2

# Chasing Quicksilver

February 1988

Silver beads puddle on the floor under my bedside table. Large and small, shiny and round. I'm on my knees, ovulation chart in one hand. As my outstretched fingers touch them, the circles shimmy away. I'm chasing quicksilver.

Before I broke it, the thermometer reported that my temperature rose today. That's good news. Yesterday, a precipitous, felicitous drop, and then today, a rise. Resurrection. On the chart, it looks like a check mark. Secret code for "I am fertile."

For a forty-year-old, divorced woman in the late 1980s, lack of a willing male partner is a fertility problem. I've been chasing the last-minute dream of having a child through artificial insemination for six months. I get the weirdness of it all: these trips to the city, the roulette of inseminations, the clinical, impersonal process of ordering up a genetic father like I was ordering an ice cream cone—three scoops, please.

But here I am. Time is running out. I drive into the city, feeling vast with possibilities. I park, enter the building, take the elevator one floor up, into the place where it will all happen. I step into the intensity of a roomful of women who have come for their babies. They glance up from their magazines.

Beyond the waiting room, in a fridge, is a vial of sperm with my name on it. The donor is anonymous, but I know he is smart and healthy. He is around six feet tall, has dark hair, and is of Eastern European or Irish lineage.

A nurse walks me to an examining room. I change and settle onto the papered, leather table. A mobile floats above me. Small, abstract shapes that weren't there last time. When the doctor arrives, chart and vial in hand, he asks what my temperature did today and begins examining me. "Your mucus looks good," he says. I smile. Radiantly. What greater compliment could there be on Day 16 of my cycle?

There's a pinch as the straw enters my cervix. All my awareness narrows to the mystery unfolding within my pelvis. Eyes closed, I am breathing the egg and the sperm into happy conjunction. This moment could change my life. Will this be the insemination that works? It could be happening.

"Do you like our new table?"

I open my eyes.

Another physician has materialized and is peering down at me. I take in the expensive, silk bowtie and the expectant grin. This must be the senior partner I haven't met. So much for the solemnity of the moment. My entire past and future are met at this instant on this table, and it doesn't matter to me what it's made of. I'm not going to discuss his leather.

He stares blankly at me for a few seconds, then vanishes like the White Rabbit.

I close my eyes and try to collect myself. My physician finishes. He makes a few notes in my chart and wishes me good luck. Everyone leaves the room, and I lie there, breathing into the beginnings of my son, Zachary.

# 3

## How I Discover Blue Sky on a Spring Morning When I Am Five Weeks Pregnant

February 1988

It is miraculous. And completely ordinary.

On the way to work, I notice the sky is blue.

Just ahead, over the Marriott Courtyard building. I blink and squint to be sure I'm not imagining it. Yes, it is blue.

Not the milky, indifferent, daily blue I've lived under for forty years. But another sky I call "vacation blue."

I'd seen it for the first time in my early thirties. Vacationing with my husband on Nantucket, free of my usual angst, I was lying in the warm sand among the dunes. I turned my head to the right and followed a rise of sand to the beginnings of dune grass, and trailed that crisp green as it rose. The tips of the grass waved like a sea of hands raised toward a god, and the god was a brilliant, infinite blue.

From then on, but only on vacation, I'd rediscover blue sky: over the snow-topped Tetons, above the high desert of New Mexico, over poppy fields in the south of France. Even England's Lake District managed a few days of vacation blue sky whenever I visited. I concluded that my world, my corner of the humid and moody East Coast, must not be able to conjure that blue. I resigned myself to that in much the same way I'd long ago accepted the overcast and narrowed world of my depression. That melancholy was a persistent, anxious, low-grade hopelessness that occasionally erupted into terror and despair. So much energy went into working around it.

But now, pregnant, nauseous, and nibbling on saltines, on an ordinary Tuesday morning in my own neighborhood, I can see that intimate, infinite blue and settle contentedly under its gaze. My new hormonal state is subtly and gently lightening my mood. I don't feel ecstatic. I feel normal, as I've always imagined others felt.

# 4

# This Tiny Life

July 1988

Half-way through my pregnancy, I know a few things about the tiny life inside me.

This baby is a boy.

He was conceived on March 3, 1988, under less than romantic circumstances.

He quickened on a sticky summer day in the Pocono Mountains as I walked up a wooden ramp into a church bazaar.

At the movies, he responds to loud soundtracks by bumping around furiously under my rib cage.

At the amniocentesis, my OB calls him "a handsome bear." My friend Tom has named him "Wrong Way Corrigan."

He prefers the breech position, with his head high on my right side. I ask him repeatedly to right himself, but he declines.

During the summer, I trade awkwardness for buoyancy and swim laps. We do it together: water all around me, me all around him in his watery sac, swimming.

His name is Zachary David.

# 5

# Still Point

November 1988

Two hours have passed since his delivery.

The hospital room is shadowy except for an overhead light that shines on us. I'm sitting up in bed. I hold on tight to a bundle that never moves and makes no sounds.

I gaze into the swaddling. Ruddy cheeks, a touch of frown across his brow, a bow mouth. All wrapped tight in a white, cotton blanket and tiny white hat. Hello, little boy.

I'm so tired. Sometimes, my eyes close and I drop into short sleeps, holding him close.

The living come and go. I know who enters the room, who must stay in the hall, who holds him, who cannot. I talk to each one who dares come close.

"Look. Here he is. Do you want to hold him? Isn't he handsome?"

Some take him in their arms and kiss his forehead.

The time will be short before the nurses take him away. They'll think me strange to want to keep him.

My therapist arrives. She stands to my right and admires my boy. We unwrap him and examine his perfect fingers and toes. Soft, soft skin.

I know there are concrete physical reasons that have caused Zachary's death. But in the clarity and madness of the moment, I am like an oracle when I turn to her and say, "This is the family script come true."

I think, but don't add, *you couldn't stop it, nor could I.*

The sadness and disconnections in the family line and in me, have converged here in this death.

She answers with silence.

I can feel the weight of generations before me. They've slipped in through the rent in time that opened with this birth. Their steps are gritty shuffles. They line the wall three deep, on the dark, far side of the room. They stand on their toes to get a look at this baby. He is the still point to which they have all come, himself a whisper of their sadness and trouble.

Great-great grandparents, and their grandparents, humble working people, hearts weakened by disappointment. Generations who learned not to want. They were good and reverent. Obedient. Silent.

Among them, other presences even I can't see. The double shades of descendants who will not be.

I hold my beautiful boy. I have him. I don't have him.

I am a banshee, a howling crack in the fabric of things. A source of horror and truth, mineral smells, and darkness.

# 6

## The Morning After

November 1988

The flat grey light at the window means day. The next day. The morning after.

This day is dangerous. It has no bottom. If I lift my head from the limp hospital pillow and dare to sit up and place my feet on the cold tile, I will evaporate. I have to be very careful.

A nurse opens the door and checks on me. I pretend to be asleep.

My curled body on the bed feels like an appendage. The real me comes and goes, sometimes huddled deep in the cave of my body, and at other times, dispersed and not exactly anywhere. I track the changing light at the window, footsteps passing in the hallway, and every sensation in my body and mind. This tracking gives me coherence. Maybe this is how I will save myself, eventually. Maybe periods of coherence will lengthen.

I look out over the frosted, barren lawn beyond my window. It stretches the length of a city block. Shrubbery edges its far end. The chill and the stark-ness soothe me.

Even after everything that has happened, the sun is about to rise. It clears the hospital building, and before disappearing into the cloud cover, reaches across the grey lawn, and ignites the shrubbery. A bush flares red. It looks like an open wound, like a womb, chaotic and alive. Terrible. Everything living surprises me.

The sound of my name draws me back. I become aware that someone is here. Betty, the nurse from my OB's practice, crouches down so that we are face to face. Many months ago, she stood beside me, touched to tears as I taped the Doppler sound of Zachary's heart beat—swish, swish, swish. Now her eyes tear up again. She leans over and hugs me. Her strength and solidity startle me. She smells freshly laundered. She already knows what has happened. But I tell her anyway. I can't not tell the story. We cry together, and she hands me five Polaroid photographs of Zachary taken the night before. There he is, swaddled and new, and so still.

For a long time after Betty leaves, I stare at the photos, trying to climb into the pictures. I want my attention to awaken him. These images are not enough, and they are everything.

I drift and doze with the pictures clenched in my hand. Time seems to pass. A friend arrives with flowers and a gift. It seems strange to bring a gift to the hospital on this day. Strange, but kind. I think I ought to open it.

The curly green ribbon offends. Too much light. Too much life. The white cardboard box feels weightless in my hands, and a small gold label reads "Bakery Shoppe." I slip off the ribbon, and side flaps rise like birds' wings. I open the box, remove a square of waxed paper, and find, on a white doily, three perfectly-formed, plump, butter cookies, and at the center of one, a thumbprint of raspberry jam.

A sharp, raw gladness slices through me. Everything has failed—God, hope, love. Everything except the brilliant, devouring, indifferent impulse to live. I see my hand reach into the box toward the glistening jam.

# 7

# A Birth Like Death

November 1988

It's a warm, November morning, the day after Thanksgiving. By a newly dug grave, I listen to familiar words.

> *...were we led all that way for*
> *Birth or Death? There was a Birth, certainly,*
> *we had evidence and no doubt. I had seen birth*
>     *and death,*
> *but had thought they were different; this Birth was*
> *hard and bitter agony for us, like Death, our*
> *death.*

Friends encircle Zachary's tiny, white coffin. Their faces are strained and sad. Some look frightened. Shrieks of horror ricochet inside me. The only way I know how to manage this moment is to wrap it in words, so I've asked a friend to read T. S. Eliot. I need the protection of the old words with their confident blending of opposites. I need their strange, soothing magic.

> *... and what you thought you came for*
> *Is only a shell, a husk of meaning*
> *From which the purpose breaks only when it is*
>     *fulfilled,*
> *If at all.*

I was sixteen and sitting in Senior English class when I first heard Eliot's words. I hadn't yet kissed a boy, or gotten my driver's license, or traveled to another country alone, but I recognized the mystery and contradiction. I had no idea what he meant, and yet I knew exactly what he meant. With Eliot, words had finally arrived in my life. They gathered me up and gave me shape. It was a birth as real as any other.

*And what the dead had no speech for, when living,*
*They can tell you, being dead....*

I've worn my favorite jade green maternity dress. It's a stylish drop-waist and doesn't look anything like the tents pregnant women used to wear. I could continue to use it even though I'm not pregnant. Of course, I won't. I can feel a light breeze rippling the fabric against my arms and legs.

*...the communication*
*of the dead is tongued with fire beyond*
*the language of the living.*

In a few minutes, I'm going to speak in the voice of a mother. I will ask my friends to remember Zachary, and to realize that in knowing me during these months, they've known him.

*And all shall be well and*
*all manner of thing shall be well.*

I want the time to go slowly. Odd to find treasure here amid this horror. I want my son, Zachary, to be honored. I want there to be an "us" just a little bit longer. The words make it so.

*We die with the dying:*
*See, they depart, and we go with them.*
*We are born with the dead....*

# 8

# Unmoored

December 1988

I had been prepared for weeks of spotty sleep, crashing hormones and the wonder of a baby boy. Instead, there is silence in the house. I spend most of my days on the sofa and prefer the curtains closed. It turns out that I am the newborn, unmoored from pregnancy and the future I'd imagined. Adrift.

Life seems terribly fragile, the world so unsafe. I'm afraid of dying myself. Death didn't just brush by. It happened inside me.

But, I keep myself alive. I make sure to eat well and exercise every day. Deep inside my grieving, without actually verbalizing it, I'm shaping a deal with a God I'm not sure I believe in. The deal goes like this: I've lost my son. There's nothing I can do about that now. I'll be good, work at recovering, and in return you will allow me another pregnancy and a healthy baby. It's only fair.

Every evening, Tom, the man I've been seeing for two years, stops on his way from work and takes me home to his house. He drops me off again at home in the morning. I exercise, then curl into the sofa, receive visits from friends, spend time with Zachary's pictures, nap, and sometimes watch television. One day, I see Bill Moyers interviewing Joseph Campbell, the Sarah Lawrence professor whose writings, research, and lectures on mythology and religion have brought him national recognition.

Campbell leans forward in his chair and tells Moyers about what he's discovered in a lifetime of world mythology studies. Myths, he says, describe the human experience, beneath all the differences of time and place and culture. Using stories about heroes and their journeys, the myths provide a roadmap. They tell us what to expect.

The hero, Campbell says, sets out on a quest, but soon learns that she is not in charge of the endeavor. She goes alone, but helpers appear. Sometimes the helpers are animals who may then turn into something else. There are terrible trials. She loses herself. Shapes shift. The hero must change her way of thinking and figure out how to hold on to her own humanity. If she persists, she finds more than she knew to hope for.

They're talking about my life. The one I am no longer in charge of.

Sitting on the sofa, I am without a belief system. Only randomness makes sense to me, and I'm not ready to give that up. But their words rearrange the emptiness.

That comforts me.

# 9

# I Am That Woman

January 1989

Here I am in a chair opposite my therapist, Catherine. Usually I lie on the leather couch, and we work analytically. Not today. I'm back, for the first time, in the room where I decided on pregnancy as a single mother. But there is no pregnancy, and no baby. Now what? I am angry with everything, including Catherine and psychology, for letting this happen to us. What can I depend on? Nothing, it seems. I refuse to make myself feel vulnerable. I slouch in the chair, and make it clear that I'm not in the mood for such make-believe as psychoanalysis.

Last week, I tried, for the sake of my friends, to brighten up, to leave the sadness and anger behind, and go out for a meal and a movie. Over a month of fractured days and nights have passed, and they thought it would do me good. They meant well. But as we moved around in the ordinary, Friday night world of the living—riding through slow traffic, crossing a busy, blacktopped parking lot, reading menus, waiting in a ticket line—I drifted away into wordless, paralyzed fog. The contrast between what had happened to us and the flow of normal life was too great. Pretending I could—or should—participate destroyed the little bit of steadiness I'd accumulated over the last weeks. I've learned my lesson: No more pretending.

I glare at Catherine, when I look at her at all. I am not going to abandon my grief and rage for her or for anyone.

I feel freed—for the first time in my life—of empathy for all the world's troubles. I like the feeling. The Lockerbie bombing has just occurred. Two hundred and fifty-nine people fell out of the sky over Scotland, and news reports talk about little else. I mention the bombing to Catherine, and shrug, "Shit happens." I mean it. I feel nothing. "Shit happens. People will have to get used to it." Grief and rage have extinguished my chronic empathy.

This rage is exquisite. Diamond-strong and clear, steady and cool. No remorse weakens it. There is no doubt or ambivalence. No fear or hope. "I've been let in on a secret that a lot of people don't know," I spit out. "Darkness is real. No amount of light can make it go away. Hard work doesn't protect us from it. Being good makes no difference. Life is a meaningless, random exercise. It's time everyone grew up."

As I spew my new credo, I think of people who do the unthinkable. I remember that story from the Old Testament about King Solomon.

As the story goes, two harlots were brought before King Solomon. Both women had recently given birth. They came before the King with one living baby between them. Each claimed the child. "No one else was in the house," said the first harlot. "It was only us. During the night, she lay on her baby and smothered him. And then she took my living child and left me her dead one."

"No!" insisted the other woman. "This living baby is mine. She is lying. It was her child who died."

King Solomon listened to the harlots, and then asked for a sword. "Cut the baby in half, and give half to each woman," he ordered. The mother of the living child begged the king to spare her baby. She would give him away rather than see him killed. But the bereaved mother said, "Divide him."

I can imagine the steel in that mother's eyes. She is a woman with nothing to lose. Grief has altered her. Her pain has uncovered the murderer in her. Of course it has.

"No one pays any attention to her when that story is told," I tell Catherine. "It's all about Solomon's wisdom. That grieving mother is just the monster who sets things in motion."

I am that woman. I, too, think it would be fair to spread the death and destruction around. I imagine causing breakage and grief that would affect thousands of people. I could bomb a subway, for instance. It won't bring my baby back, but it would give voice to my long, silent scream.

I leave our session thinking about that bible story. The mother with the living baby went home, but what about the other harlot? The bereaved, half-mad mother. Did she disappear into the desert and wait there to die? Did she roam the dusty streets wailing her grief and her rage? Was she stoned for stealing another woman's child?

If Solomon really were wise, if his consciousness were evolved enough, this is how the story would have ended:

> The King held the grieving mother in his arms. He ordered his favorite wife to take her, bathe and anoint and dress her, and sit with her to talk about the lost child. "What was his name?" "Did he resemble you?" "Did you labor long?" "Did he cry easily?" "Sleep a lot?"
>
> The King's wife watched over the harlot who ate and slept and mourned in the palace for a long time. Each day they walked on the palace terraces where they spoke the boy's name onto the dry, sweet breezes that blew there. The harlot grew strong and calm, and when she was at last ready, she found her way back.

# 10

## The Shortest Story

May, 1989

I've never doubted that I will try again to become pregnant. Wanting another chance has been a twin preoccupation to my grieving for Zachary. I've longed for the cry of a healthy, living baby to soften his silence.

I return to the fertility practice for inseminations. A hopeful wariness has replaced the innocent excitement I used to feel. I know what happens next is out of my control. In two months, I greet the news of my pregnancy like a widow who is still wearing black but is curious about the suitor waiting in the parlor.

From the beginning, my hormone count is sluggish. I don't particularly feel pregnant, but my physician and I want to hope. At the end of six weeks, she calls the pregnancy a blighted ovum. The fertilized egg that found its way to the uterine wall and settled in is long gone. The sac that will never be a placenta continues to pump hormones into its emptiness.

My distress is so diffuse and turbulent that I can't focus to mourn. I'm horrified that nature can be so cavalier, giving life and allowing it to end indiscriminately in humans as much as in gardens, galaxies, or animals. What I've already lost and suffered doesn't actually matter. I don't get a free pass, even though

I've been a good girl. I only get to be part of life. At this moment, that's not enough.

My physician explains that eventually, my body will stop supporting the sac and it will pass as blood and clots. It feels impossible to carry the emptiness any longer. I have a D & C, and it is over.

# 11

# Things Worse Than Death

June 1989

Early on, my grief felt like a buffering fog. I walked slower, thought slower, drifted away if a conversation exceeded a few paragraphs. At times, unstoppable weeping possessed me. Fear and panic, deep sadness and anger came and went. I was softened and laid low, transformed into a walking, talking shadow. And there was nothing I could do about it. Any attempt to "put on a happy face" felt harrowing, like my soul was being plucked from me.

Grief brought heightened awareness of myself, mind and body, and in that way, it was busy, organic, and full. It didn't separate me from myself the way depression had. In fact, it was oddly companionable. I was suffering terribly, but I was enclosed and protected, and somehow, still connected to life. That early fog kept reality at a manageable distance

That has all changed. My miscarriage has voided the deal I made with God. Grief, rage, and bitterness saturate me.

Two pregnancies have failed. I am alone, again, with nothing to show for my efforts. My friends are supportive, but exhausted. I distinctly feel a hole in my heart, and I've been wearing a square of red silk under my clothes and in front of my heart to shield it. That deep red is also my private, emphatic assertion that I have had enough. I wouldn't have thought it possible that I could be angrier than I was after Zachary died. But I am. No foggy buffer this time. I am done with bravery, hope and patience.

My private psychotherapy practice is still small enough that I can bundle my appointments in the middle of the week and escape my own chaos on long weekends. I've gone to a couple of conferences and retreats, and run away to New England and out to Nantucket. With each arrival, I've hoped my agitation would subside, but these places I once loved feel cold and menacing.

My old depression is returning with its terrors and distorted beliefs, those remnants of my child-self's explanations about why things go wrong: *I can't make a life as others do. I'm not good enough. I'm odd, different, defective, forgotten.* That depressive narrative brings me into a deeper, more dangerous darkness than grief has. Everything is impossibly difficult.

A good friend is away on vacation. I know I can get into her garage, and that is where I'd do it. I'd drive in, close the door behind me, turn on the engine and be done. I can picture the brown panels on that garage door.

I tell myself I haven't done it because I don't want to hurt my friend. She would return and find me, and that is no way to repay her many kindnesses.

If I were determined to die, I'd have plan B and C in place. I don't. These suicidal thoughts comfort me because they promise a way out when there is none.

# 12

## Being Body

August 1989

Before pregnancy, I had a body. Being pregnant,
I became a body. And for nine months, through
nausea and the end of nausea, through shape-shifting,
heightened sensuality, hormonal glow, shifting moods,
exhaustion, and Zachary's bumps and flutters, I lived
in almost constant awareness of and amazement at
my resourceful, vividly alive body. The sensation of
my uterus emptying at delivery felt like a final exhale.
After that, my body seemed to darken and drift away.
I lost touch with it, except for that sense of emptiness.
I fed it because I had to if I were ever going to have
another child. I exercised it for the same reason. The
miscarriage has completed the estrangement.

Now my body feels distant except when anxiety
or anger agitate it and remind me of my own physical
presence. I've had some digestive problems. For a
while, swallowing was incredibly painful, as if I were
swallowing sharp knives. And there've been cramping,
vague aches and fatigue. My body has failed me not
once but twice.

A friend has suggested an acupressure session as
a comforting way to support my body in its grieving.
She explains that acupressure is similar to acupuncture in that it restores the balance of energy flows
in the body and is known to reduce muscle tension
and fatigue, improve the workings of the lymphatic

system, and release emotion. Acupressure uses light pressure instead of needles, along the meridians or energy flow lines that run vertically on the body, front and back.

I accept her generous offer and have my first experience of energy work. Wearing everyday clothes, I lay in her office on a massage table. Soft music plays. The wordlessness of the treatment appeals to me. I've lost confidence in talking things through so I am happy to lie down and be still.

She moves around the table, holding points on various meridian lines. Lying there soothes me, and for a while, nothing else happens. Then I begin to feel occasional sensations, like breaths, or like a ruffling movement inside my leg, through my chest, and down my spine.

Like everyone, I want my body to function smoothly and to look good. The same expectations you'd have toward a really reliable limousine. Get me where I want to go and don't confuse me with all that scary stuff under the hood. Oh, and please be shiny.

Occasionally, before my pregnancy experiences, I'd notice my body's aliveness when I felt my heart beat or watched my menstrual cycle come and go, or enjoyed my sensuality. But mostly, I saw my body as a tool that made my life possible.

The sensations I experience on the massage table awaken me to a subtler aspect of my being. I am present and embodied. I feel more whole, and less alone. These subtle flows of energy remind me of the sensations of pregnancy. But what I'm feeling isn't another life. It is mine. I am meeting my own deeper being.

The acupuncture session is another birth for me, and a great gift. As I experience the subtle energy within me, I feel deep compassion for myself and a new sense of tenderness. The kind of patient, open-heartedness I try to give to others I can feel for myself. It is like meeting my body's own vast life. The wonder of simply being touches me. It goes beyond happy or sad and doesn't depend on what is going on around me. In its presence, stories fade. I find I exist in an aliveness more enveloping than I ever imagined.

I leave the session feeling part flesh and blood, and part steady, luminous light.

# 13

# Letting Go

October 1989

I tell my clients that the nature of emotion is to be fluid. It comes. It goes. But, sometimes an emotion will come, settle into the bodymind and stay. That's what has happened with my anger and discouragement about the miscarriage. Months of therapy, bodywork, and writing have offered relief and given me the beginnings of a new normal, but I am still preoccupied with the injustice of it, and my body is complaining, too, with persistent intestinal problems.

A friend suggested performing a ritual for letting go in which we would share readings, listen to music, examine the subject of loss and letting go, and use gestures and symbols that say we're willing to let go of our losses and our suffering over them.

I've been ambivalent about doing the ritual. While I do believe that focused, communal reflection and gesture can create change, I'm hesitant to have us assume the role of actually officiating at a ceremony we design. In my world, priests and other anointed people lead rituals. What gives us the authority? And besides, maybe it's just New Age woo-woo. Doing a ritual would mean we are either subversive or flakey, and neither of those is appealing.

I'm surprised to see my hesitation since I thought I believed that we are all naturally plugged in to the divine or whatever you want to call it. I'm even more surprised to admit that I'm a little afraid it will actually work! Do I want to acknowledge we all have the power to change and heal? Wouldn't that be having too much power?

But the idea of ritual warms my heart. I'm going ahead with the ceremony because it will be comforting not to be alone with my emotions.

Doing the ritual outdoors feels right, so two friends and I spread a blanket on a hillside at Valley Forge Park. Our spot overlooks a rolling expanse of tall, coarse grass just beginning to turn from green to yellow. All around us, an ordinary autumn Sunday unfolds. On the road that passes about ten yards from us, bikers sail by, leaning into the air. Visitors stop their cars to read inscriptions on the monuments. Families walk dogs, and couples hold hands as they pass.

The objects scattered on our blanket are not the usual picnic gear: votive lights, rocks, feathers, a CD player, poetry books, sage burning in a sturdy sea shell. It feels strange and appropriate to be doing a ritual in the midst of such ordinariness.

Sitting together in the breezy sunlight, we revisit our losses, cry and laugh, and share stories. We allow difficult emotions to be present as we talk about experiences of letting go, not wanting to let go, being let go of. Each of us shares a reading on the subject. We listen to flute music and meditate. Our square of blanket offers comfort and security.

Earlier in the week, a friend gave me a bird's feather she'd found. She said it reminded her of my miscarriage. It is white and tiny, barely half an inch, the kind of soft, downy feather that lies hidden beneath other feathers, close to the bird's body. It helps keep the bird warm.

When I feel ready, I stand up, remove the feather from its matchstick box, and place it in the palm of my hand. As the breeze lifts the feather from my outstretched hand, I'm sad and a little frightened, but also comforted by the sensation of the warm, calm breeze. I see I am relinquishing the feather and my losses to another, larger kind of life.

That simple gesture begins to break down the isolation I've been feeling. Letting go is as much a beginning as an ending. Maybe, like the feather, I can move ahead into the future.

I come away feeling emotionally lighter, and my cramping and intestinal troubles end shortly after.

# 14

# Motherhood

February 1990

I am forty-two years old. Time is running out.

Most parents will go on to have a successful pregnancy after a stillbirth. My miscarriage a few months after Zachary derailed my efforts to conceive again, and nearly a year has passed. It was a hard, dark year and I am grateful to have survived it. I'm grateful too for the beginnings of a spiritual life and a warmer and more conscious relationship with my body. Both resources give me a sense of grounding and sturdiness that I didn't have before. And I am very, very thankful for the antidepressant I now take.

I've wanted to try again, though the prospect of another pregnancy frightens me. I know what can go wrong. How will I manage the terror? When I try to imagine a successful delivery, my mind can only replay Zachary's birth. I've told my friends I'm resuming inseminations, and that is when the frightening dreams begin. They come regularly, at night and even during naps. Dream after dream of being trapped, deeply depressed, and unloved.

Side effects of the drug Clomid, used to stimulate follicle growth, are a challenge on a good day, and now they add another layer of emotional stress. Mood shifts and fatigue weight my days. As the inseminations begin, I develop a self-care routine that includes daily naps, very little sugar, meditation, baths, relaxations, journal writing, and avoidance of people and events that tax me. Even so, I often have headaches and feel flu-ish in addition to daytime anxiety and the unnerving dreams.

In spite of all my self-care, I am physically and emotionally exhausted. The dreams and the physical stress symptoms continue. The fertility specialists are now using frozen sperm, which decreases the success rate. I've had to stop using antidepressants, and I am losing the struggle to maintain my newfound steadiness. I am in the midst of a new relationship, but it is much too early to know how that will unfold. I still expect to be a single mother.

I've seen women muster extraordinary courage to undertake a pregnancy after loss. And sometimes their odds of being successful were not as good as mine. Many keep at it at great cost to themselves and their partners until they have a healthy birth. After three months of inseminations, it has become clear to me that I can't do that.

I have felt like I am entering a danger zone. If I knew other ways to manage the trauma, I might find a way to go on. But I don't. I am so, so tired. I decide to preserve myself. I stop the inseminations, and the relief is immediate. The dreams stop.

In the months that follow, it is not the next pregnancy I grieve. It is my motherhood, that identity I'd inhabited with Zachary: fierce, tender, excited, frightened, fulfilled, intimate, constant, and constantly changing. My pregnancy motherhood was a clear identifier. This is who I am. This is who we are. We are family. Going on now without a living child, I don't appear to be a mother. And in relinquishing my public motherhood, I'm giving up Zachary again. It will be harder to keep his name alive without being engaged in the world of young children. He won't live on as the older brother to be spoken of and remembered.

One grief seems to give birth to another. They're only manageable because stopping feels as right as the original choice to try.

# 15

# Bereaved Clients

January 1991

My obstetrician has begun sending me bereaved parents for counseling. It's been a couple of years, and the prospect of working with them both pleases and frightens me. I don't know if I can be in the presence of that particular kind of pain and still be useful. Will their suffering ignite my own sadness and overwhelm me? Helping grieving parents will challenge all my theories about maintaining clinical distance with clients. I don't know if I can do it, but I want to try.

In my twenties and thirties, I'd experienced a rash of family deaths including my parents. Most were unexpected, some devastating. I saw how those losses upended and rearranged our lives and couldn't escape learning what made grief bearable and what slowed it down, as well as the high cost of trying to avoid it. Grief hurt, and at times felt disabling, but it followed a predictable course, and it had an end. In retrospect, it seemed like a time outside of time full of potential for change. I decided that somewhere in my career as a psychologist, I'd like to work with people in mourning. I never dreamed how that would come about.

The first client is a young mother who had a stillbirth six weeks earlier. When I greet her in the waiting room, I see eyes lost in a drawn, blank facial mask, just edged with panic. She is a woman with just enough strength to stay alert for the next disaster that must surely be coming her way. I know that state of mind and soul, and I feel that terrible despondency again.

We begin to talk and my client describes the routine checkup that turned into heartbreak. She revisits the delivery, her family's time with her daughter, the burial and then the endless, empty hours and days that follow. Talking about Michelle, her daughter, brings tears to her eyes and a spark of life to her weary face. Already, she explains, there are few opportunities to say Michelle's name aloud or to tell her story. Yet I can see that this very simple telling breathes life into my client. I ask if she has a picture. She slips one out of her wallet and presents it to me. Now, there are no tears, just fierce pride.

She fears that she is going crazy. Isolated in her grief and anxiety, she needs to know what is normal. Everyone is worried about her, she says. We talk about the wide band of what is normal grief, and I help her identify what soothes her suffering, and who she can count on to let her go through this at her own pace.

Afterward, I think about the session and how it felt to sit with my client. I know this territory. I know the feel of madness threatening, the disorientation and hollowness and isolation. But what strikes me most is this: I am surprised that stillbirth is still happening. She has reminded me that every day families are still hearing some version of those terrible words, "We can't find a heartbeat." Unconsciously, I have been pretending that this kind of calamity ended after Zachary died. That the world has become a safe place again. I know that makes no sense, but the magical thinking connected with grief and trauma is inescapable. Working with grieving parents will mean facing the fact that the unthinkable does continue to happen.

I have met with many bereaved parents since that day with Michelle's mother. I've loved being of service to them. When it seems appropriate, I share my own experience. It seems to comfort them that I know their situation first hand. On occasion, their stories activate my trauma and sadness and I have to take care to soothe and refresh myself afterward. But I do love working with them.

These parents come with pain and pride in the babies they've lost. They bring photos, trauma-seared memories, and the nearly universal questions, "What did I do wrong?" and "Am I going crazy?" They all report a nagging sense that the world wants them to shut up and move on.

Their sessions honor their lost children. I teach them about grief and how to ride it out. In a way, I stand for the future, theirs and their families. It's a future that includes their deceased child in ways we can't yet predict. It can also include the enriched selves they are becoming by mourning their children.

I relearn in these sessions that grief is the most idiosyncratic of emotions. No two people do it the same way. And I'm reminded that grief attended to moves on, though it never, never feels like it will.

# 16

# Nothing Pink About It

May 1992

Forget the flowers
forget the sentimental cards

Mothers' Day honors
deep earth potency

Think fierce blood-red
relentless spring green
new moon darkness

Celebrate
vast unruly urges
sprouts thrusting toward light
the devouring yawn of a quake

Understand this
Mothers give life
voluptuous
unpredictable
chaotic

There's nothing pink about it

# 17

# The Thing That is Hoped For

April 1993

I'm lying on the sofa, watching the afternoon light fill the living room, enjoying the post-massage sensation of my entire body breathing.

A mineral scent encircles me.

*All slate and talc, broad, gentle, no sharp edges, no flower or spice. Elemental. Deep earth.*

Though it's been over five years, I know Zachary's scent. I actually sit up and look around, expecting to see him.

*Suddenly, we are together again. Then is now. There is here. We are together. We. We are.*

I float in his mineral scent. I want to inhale him, and then hold my breath to keep him with me.

*I can feel the softness of his body and see the dim quiet of the delivery room.*

*Stay. Stay.*

In less than a minute, the scent begins to fade. He's leaving. Again.

I lay still for a long while, stunned and grateful and hoping he will return. When he doesn't, I call my practitioner and ask if she'd used any oils that could have created this scent. She says she had not, but has known bodies to release memory through scent.

How can such an extraordinary experience come and go so quietly? Where and how, I wonder, along the great continuum of living things, does memory cross over into the very fine matter of scent molecules? Where and how do memory and matter become presence? And how do I understand the way in which time and place merged while his scent hovered?

I can accept that the body releases scent but along with that, I know I've had an emotional, even spiritual encounter. Connection is multilayered.

My encounter reminds me of a phenomenon that occurs during pregnancy in which fetal cells cross the placenta and migrate into the mother. They can exist in her tissues and organs for decades. The fetal cells that stay are called microchimera. In ancient cosmologies, a chimera was a mythic animal made from parts of various other animals. We all are chimera, made up of parts of others. Zachary's DNA probably lives in me today. That too is an encounter.

The word "chimera" also means "the thing that is hoped for but illusory." In more ways than I ever imagined, my hoped-for, illusory child and I are part of each other. That pleases me.

# 18

# The Gods We Choose Decide Everything About Us

August 1995

Zachary's death has forced me to re-examine my ideas about how life works. What's the point of it all? What do I believe in? How do I fit this saddest of deaths into a world view and a spirituality that makes sense to me?

Even before Zachary, I'd given up on the God of my childhood and had come to believe only in the randomness of things. Not having a God to be disappointed in, or to argue with, simplified my grief. Zachary's death and the miscarriage came as more data confirming that anything bad can happen to anybody, anytime. I'd been caught at the dark edge of the odds.

But my randomness philosophy isn't holding up. While the world I live in certainly brims with the haphazard, there is also so much order. So much connection among parts. I think my randomness theory fails primarily because it's about disconnection. Over these years since Zachary, the work I've done to survive has had the collective effect of bringing me into many connections: with myself and my body, with subtle energies and a spiritual realm, with new friends and pursuits, and new ways of approaching my work. I can't deny that.

I want to be clear now that the spirituality I adopt matches what I've come to know in my gut. It has to spring from inside me, develop from experience, not doctrine, and it has to be able to hold contradictions.

I've wandered from Quakers to Buddhists to Unitarians, trying to find a spiritual home. Each system has nourished me in its way, but none has felt like home. As I search, I am repeatedly drawn back to the very simple, basic ideas Joseph Campbell gleaned from his studies in mythology and world religions. In those interviews I watched during my maternity leave, he talked about many gods, about the universal impulse to seek and believe and transcend that led all peoples to their own forms of connection with the divine. As I recall his description of humanity's spiritual history, I can see a spiritual attitude capable of containing the chaos of life. One that includes and honors the inevitable cycles of life and death, light and dark, knowing and not knowing. In this worldview, nothing is static. Life sprawls forward. Good things happen, horrible things happen. It's all life. Anchored to nature's rhythms, humans learned to live in a more-than-human and less-than-human world. Maybe I can survive that way, too.

I feel embraced and comforted by the wish to exist consciously within a larger order of life. I'm beginning to understand that connection, continuity and being part of the flow of life are at the heart of spirituality. This developing spirituality can encompass the wonder of a baby as well as the horror of his death. Without narrowing the divine down to a single god, I can believe in an infinite intelligence that is everywhere and of which I am a part.

That's what I know so far.

# 19

## Then I Have a Dream

December 1996

Eight years have passed since Zachary. From the outside, my life looks great. I move from the office to get-togethers with friends, to dates and holidays, to writing, to time at home alone, and I enjoy each in itself. But my days and weeks feel like a series of short hops. They aren't adding up to a life.

My past doesn't accumulate. It vanishes behind me like a jet trail. Since college there've been several try-outs at careers, marriage and later, a divorce; a move, graduate school, settling into my psychology career, another move, Zachary's death and the miscarriage. My parents are gone, and my only sibling and his family live a life abroad that makes connection between us difficult. My favorite aunt and uncle are also dead. I hadn't expected to be alone this long after my divorce, and I envy friends whose lives have unfolded more conventionally, from college to career, marriage and family. Though pregnancy and antidepressants and doing work I love have opened up a broader, happier life for me, I feel a lingering sense of disconnection. I've run out of ideas about how to fix it.

And then, I have a dream.

I am marooned in an airport, unable to get confirmed on a flight home when a dog, a greyhound, crosses the terminal, sits beside me and reminds me that I don't have to remain there waiting for a turn that never comes. She adds that there is a world of other things to do.

I feel wonder and sweet relief at having her beside me. She warms my heart and soothes that chronic futility.

Dreams have become an important part of my life. While working with a Jungian Analyst, I've learned they are a source of revelation I can trust to correct and round out the narrower viewpoint of waking consciousness. The point of this dream isn't to tell me to get a greyhound. That would be too literal. The elegant greyhound image is developing into a nourishing presence in my psyche.

She is the unexpected and instinctive in the midst of schedules and machinery. She makes me feel chosen. She suggests there are unthought-of options. The futility of standing in unmoving lines may not be my fate. Something different is possible. She knows things I don't, in ways that I haven't yet learned to know. I'm glad she's found me.

# 20

## Homecoming

March 1997

In the years after Zachary died and I decided not to try another pregnancy, I did consider adoption. I consulted parents who had adopted, and even attended a conference on open adoptions. But it never seemed right for me. I let the idea idle in the back of my mind, though. I had another ten years in which I could qualify if I chose to adopt.

It's turning out that there is an adoption, however it's one I had never anticipated.

The dream of the greyhound continues to work in me and her image keeps its freshness. I still laugh to myself at the irony of a greyhound in an airport. My connection to her is breathing new hope into my thoughts for the future.

I've been curious and have been researching the breed. That has led to reading everything I can find about greyhounds as pets. My behavior puzzles me because I've come from a long line of dog-free people who could never understand why adults took on the extra responsibilities of pets. I already live with two cats. That should be enough.

But I've begun to recall how much I'd wanted a dog as a child, how I loved visiting my uncle's dog, Blackie. I envied the bond I saw between them. And I envied the intelligence and freedom Blackie radiated as he went about his dog life. Why has it never occurred to me to have a dog of my own? Maybe I've been too driven and too practical. What else have I forgotten I wanted?

Much to my surprise, I am adopting a greyhound. This new adventure has brought me around again to that zone between longing and terror that preceded my decision to get pregnant. Can I do this? Do I have the patience and generosity? What if I resent the responsibility? What if I can't love or aren't loved? I don't want to be drawn, then disappointed.

As I prepare the house and office, I wait for a call from the rescue organization telling me that the greyhound chosen for me has died in his sleep, or been killed in a fight with another dog, or got loose and was run over. And even if he does arrive, I fear we won't bond. I just can't picture this working.

Two weeks after applying, I go the greyhound kennel to pick up a young hound. I requested a two-year-old, male greyhound with black and grey brindle markings. But when a vet tech hands me the neon orange leash, I find on the other end not the dog I'd asked for but a four-year-old, red brindle female who looks exactly like the greyhound in my dream. For a few seconds, the distinction between waking and dreaming evaporates, and I'm standing in both worlds at once.

Everything I know about dogs I've learned from books. All the unanswered questions remain. But as I walk TwylaRose to the car, deep pleasure and excitement overwhelm me. She is here and healthy. Nothing bad has happened. I am amazed.

I am engaged in something bigger than adopting a pet. We arrive home and I feel like I am watching us from a few steps away. As I see myself lead TwylaRose from the car to the front door, the shadows of that other homecoming begin to part like an observatory dome that opens to reveal a larger, brighter universe.

# 21

# Walking TwylaRose

September 1997

I walk TwylaRose four times day in all kinds of weather, and much to my surprise, I love it. For her, every walk is a grand adventure. Watching her discover her surroundings awakens me to the beauty and diversity of life just beyond my front door.

I see what I'd been rushing by in my daily busyness: the mauve of slow forming pine cones, new spring grass, the varieties of sky blue, night woods lit with fireflies, chicory and day lilies at the edge of a path. The rhythm of our days is now built around our walks. I think I enjoy them as much as she does.

It turns out I've joined a lively community of neighborhood dog people, and each walk brings greetings and friendly small talk. Three of these encounters lead to important friendships with women who also have greyhounds. Our hounds become The Pack: Ike, Christa, Pepper, and TwylaRose, and we grow into an extended family who gathers for spontaneous suppers and celebrates holidays and birthdays, always in the company of four greyhounds who at any moment might be milling or sleeping or racing in the yard.

# 22

# Disclaimer

July 1998

I didn't adopt a greyhound as a substitute for a child. To prove this, I make sure never to refer to myself as TwylaRose's mother. When others do, I ignore it. I want that part of my life to have nothing to do with this part.

I try to limit my baby talk to her and keep the number of affectionate nicknames to a minimum. This is difficult.

When others comment on the winter coat I've sewn for her—it is a blue-green polar fleece print with a matching snood—I point out that greyhounds have thin hair and no body fat and are very sensitive to the cold. Therefore, she has to have a coat.

In the winter months, I tuck a light blanket around her at night. Again, no body fat, thin hair. It is the least I can do.

The truth is that my efforts to contain this relationship in the human-pet category are being overwhelmed by a vast "I love TwylaRose" part of me. I imagine new neural pathways forming in my brain as I walk beside her or feel her warm lean on my leg. The mothering in me is awakening whole. Not only can I do this, but I love taking care of her, playing with her, and getting to know her. I'd always worried that I wouldn't be able to put another being first. I'd questioned whether I would be a good-enough mother. In our time together, I'm finding patience and generosity in myself that I'd doubted. Savoring the joyous aspects of my mother-self actually connects me back to my son. I am caring for TwylaRose, but I am also experiencing myself as I would have been with Zachary.

After an infant loss, life can find us again. In my case, that meant a retired racer, her three friends, and the humans who came with them. I don't think of that now as substituting one love for another or leaving my son behind. I think we allow life, not in place of the loved one but in place of that death. The loved one is woven into us.

# 23

# The Scent of Grief

May 1999

My new client's daughter was stillborn very recently.

When the client arrives, late, she barely says hello, drifts into my office and sits on the sofa.

Clients usually comment on the greyhound asleep in the corner. But Lily, as I'll call her, simply knots her hands in her lap and stares at the floor, as if she'd used up all her strength getting herself here. I ask her to tell me the story of her loss.

She rouses herself just enough to speak. It was a much wanted pregnancy with unexpected problems at delivery and an emergency C-section that came too late. Her daughter, Teresa, is gone. As Lily speaks, an occasional tear escapes down her cheek.

I breath slowly and consciously to stay centered as the quality of her grief becomes clearer. There are griefs that loom and taunt, swollen by their accumulated, unrelieved energy. It's as if there is no release valve to allow the emotions to come and go, to peak and quiet down again. This is that kind of grief.

I am concerned. Nothing is moving here. Lily continues, caught in the stupor-like grip of her mourning. "I can see my daughter's grave when I stand at the living room window. The cemetery is across the street."

I'm taking in the enormity of her pain when just then, TwylaRose steps off her bed and crosses the room. She stands close to Lily, sniffs her, and licks a tear from her cheek. Lily closes her eyes and begins to sob. TwylaRose goes back to her bed.

I wait. As Lily weeps, her grief unfreezes a bit. Life, painful but vital, flows again. We talk for a while longer.

I wish TwylaRose had been here when I was grieving Zachary.

# 24

# Like a Porcelain Cup and Saucer

October 2000

I've been asked to address a group of obstetricians on the psychological effects of complicated deliveries and pregnancy losses among their patients. As I prepare, I suspect they'd heard it all before.

What I need is a metaphor, an image that will deepen their understanding of what they know intellectually. It would help to have an object they could actually touch, one that captures the state of traumatized and grieving parents and allows the docs to experience their responses to their patients' needs.

I have a large set of porcelain china that I dearly love. German-made, it is white with hand-painted flowers. I try to use the bowl with the orange tulip on the bottom whenever I can, and I never tire of seeing that tulip glow up at me as I finish eating. If I hold a cup up to a sunny window, the porcelain looks translucent. On the day of my talk to the OB's, I pack up one cup and saucer to take along.

Once I've covered the basics required for their continuing education credits, I put aside the handouts and the magic marker. I unwrap the porcelain cup and saucer and hold it up in the late afternoon light.

"This is what I imagine, what I've experienced, a grieving parent feels like. Fragile, transparent, vulnerable. And of course, unique." They watch and nod.

I hand the porcelain to a physician in the front row and ask him to touch it and examine it and to then pass it on to his colleague. I watch as the cup and saucer move from hand to hand. An attentive silence falls over the room. The physicians are so careful. Some express concern that they might break it. One doc asked why I would bring something so valuable and fragile and allow everyone to touch it.

And that, of course is my point. Afterward, I share that I did feel a bit anxious as my porcelain was handed around. It is of great value to me, and I'd surrendered it to them. Also, I say I am touched by the intense relationship I observed between the docs and the cup and saucer. They admired their beauty, recognized their value, and felt some anxiety about keeping them safe as the pieces passed through their hands.

In pregnancy, and at delivery, especially when there are complications, parents and infants are as vulnerable as fine porcelain. And more valuable.

# 25

# A Good Death

December 2001

When my first greyhound, TwylaRose, is diagnosed with bone cancer and given two months to live, I wonder how I will face another death. But my experience with her death is different from any I've had before.

Once beyond the initial shock, sadness, and a couple of weeks of nausea, I begin to be drawn into her dying process. The coming separation intensifies every hour. Maybe that heightened mindfulness expands my ordinary consciousness, or maybe knowing death is imminent activates other ways of seeing and knowing that lie dormant in our rational day-to-day selves. In any case, it feels like a veil between the worlds is thinning. It becomes easier to see beyond the visible, material world and relax into my more intuitive, receptive mind. Away from TwylaRose one day, I feel the spontaneous sensation of a hug, and I know it is her enclosing me in what I'd have to call love.

I help each client say goodbye in her and his own way. One uses an animal communicator—essentially a psychic who facilitates conversations between humans and animals. In that goodbye talk, the communicator describes TwylaRose advising the client to remember that she is a good person and should, metaphorically speaking, avoid looking in mirrors that give her a distorted picture of who she is. Several nights later, the wire holding a mirror over my fireplace fails after hanging there for years. The old, oval mirror clatters to the slate floor. I give it, unbroken, to my client.

As Twyla declines, I think of Zachary frequently. The unexpectedness of his death added a layer of trauma to my grief and precluded any chance of participating in his dying. Being with TwylaRose through her last months is healing some of that trauma.

The time with her reminds me that there is a bigger, deeper life where boundaries are fluid and possibilities are abundant. In this more than ordinary consciousness, everything and everyone are somehow connected. I've had other experiences of this more spacious life, but it has always been hard to admit that yes, this is real.

If I accept the existence of this larger consciousness, it follows that I will always have a relationship with Zachary. Yet I still am afraid. I can allow that an ongoing connection exists with Twyla and with some deceased family and friends. But not Zachary. A connection to him is something I want too much to admit, or to trust is possible. So, in a way, I keep him at a distance.

When I say that being with TwylaRose during her dying is healing, I don't mean that it is always easy. Her pain becomes unmanageable, as the vet had warned it would, and my greyhound friends and I take her to be euthanized on the evening of the day after Christmas. We all grieve her terribly. A couple of weeks later, I come down with severe bronchitis and have to go to one friend's house to sleep and be cared for.

# 26

# Getting Over It

February 2002

Though these are the words that are used, "getting over it" isn't the best way to describe recovery from a loss like stillbirth. You get over mumps or the fear of snarling, black dogs. My life since Zachary has been more paradoxical, more like a series of round-abouts and switchbacks that often bears no resemblance to forward progress. Somewhere in the journey healing begins.

Here's what "getting over it" looks like for me.

Staying in bed in a darkened room and not answering the phone. Losing friends, really good friends, who think it should be otherwise.

Staring at Zachary's pictures. Putting the negatives in a safe deposit box. Having a portrait sketched from one of those pictures. Feeling proud of his handsomeness.

Hating all pregnant women.

Noticing my brisk stride is returning.

Finding new friends.

Going out to socialize, but needing to come home early and be quiet.

Hearing myself laugh for the first time in a long time.

Raging in a support group when a woman says death is an illusion. Disagreeing bitterly and loudly.

Going away for a long weekend without having a panic attack.

Having lightning strike moments like this. I'm clearing the table after supper and a conviction takes abrupt and complete possession of me: if I'd chosen to have Zachary turned out of his breech position, we could have saved him. I could have saved him. I want to call my OB and berate him.

Giving a speech to bereaved parents about miscarriage and feeling vulnerable and invulnerable all at once.

Feeling less alone than I ever have.

Giving away his baby clothes.

Surviving a breakup. Later, beginning a new relationship, my first post-Zachary, and finding that there's very little that is life-or-death important.

Realizing halfway through one Mothers' Day that I am wearing a t-shirt that says "Shit happens."

Visiting a friend post-surgery. He happens to be on the same floor as maternity at the hospital where I delivered. My stomach drops, my knees get shaky, and my breath goes shallow.

Beginning to entertain again.

Feeling angry and terrified when a client mentions a stillbirth of forty years ago and insists that "you never get over it."

Beginning a meditation practice.

Feeling comfortable and sad and useful with clients who've lost children.

Taking off the day of Zachary's anniversary and remembering our time together.

Almost forgetting the approach of his anniversary.

Seeing friends' children graduate from college, and wondering why I don't think about him more, or feel connected to him.

Considering selling the grave I bought when Zachary died. I'll be cremated and won't need it. Thinking I'd have his remains disinterred and cremated to be scattered with me. And never quite getting around to it.

Driving in the city, passing under a crane that is moving a large slab of marble over the street, I panic: it will certainly fall on me. Even good odds are problematic now. I detour to avoid it.

Having days and weeks pass when nobody dies and nothing bad happens.

Reading about the availability of Chinese children for adoption and feeling the old, urgent, wish for a child. Being sad when it passes.

Tensing up when newly pregnant women assume they'll have successful deliveries.

Listening as a friend's husband says he envies my child-free life, and realizing I'm very contented in it.

Beginning my tradition of Christmas Eve celebrations. I watch a chubby baby crawl across the room and settle under my greyhound who remains standing quietly over him. Beautiful.

# 27

## Sound

October 2003

When I think of Zachary's silence at birth, I imagine myself standing in the second floor hallway of the house where I grew up. I call to him, and call again. No response comes. The empty silence harrows the air.

That may be why I don't mind hearing babies cry. In the supermarket or on the street, or at home when friends bring their little ones, my ears perk up and absorb the pitch and timbre of baby sounds. I let their screams and whimpers play through my skin and bones and nervous system like breeze drifting through summer linen. Their sounds enliven dense spots of stillbirth silence that linger in my cells.

Recently, a client has been bringing her four-month-old girl to the office. She and I have worked together since before her pregnancy. When Pearl arrived a mellow, second child, we wondered if she would recognize my voice. When she's restless during a session, I offer to hold her.

I lay her in my lap and we sound back and forth. Grunts, gurgles, whines, cries, sighs. I think we both enjoy it.

# 28

# Writer

May 2005

I'd bought a pretty, green, marbled book to record Zachary's first days. After he died, I didn't want to fill that book with darkness so I didn't use it. But I did need to write. A friend brought me a simple, spiral-bound notebook. Writing in it saved my life.

The simple act of holding a pen and releasing words onto the paper helped me grasp what was happening during the days after his death: Zachary, stillbirth, mother, death, autopsy, funeral, frightened. Writing is different than saying the words out loud. Something about running words through my fingers gives me the distance I need to stay connected to the moment. Even if I can't stop the story, I can slow it down on paper.

I have always wanted to write, but other than my doctoral dissertation, an occasional poem, and a few freelance interviews for the local newspaper, I haven't. Since Zachary, I've written pieces about us for the newsletter of the support group, UNITE. Joining other parents in that newsletter as they give voice to their children's names and stories has been so healing. I will always appreciate their welcoming kindness.

Now, I can't imagine not writing. I've published a chapbook of poetry. A bit of fiction, essays, and poetry have been picked up by anthologies, newspapers, and magazines. I've finished a book on dreams that will be published in 2006. More important, I've gotten to experience the magic by which writing unfolds an idea far beyond my original thought. I love riding the creative process and learning to use the power of language. Writing has instilled an order into my life that deeply satisfies me. It's also brought me dear friends and generous teachers.

I am most alive when I am writing. There's nothing like it. It's the sweetest of the gifts of Zachary's life.

# 29

# Appropriately Inappropriate

September 2007

On the morning of my sixty-fifth birthday, in an unusual act of rebellion, my greyhounds escape the house. Lilith sees the open front door, seizes the moment, and shoots out onto the lane. Strider, the homebody of the pair follows, though he does throw a glance at me over his shoulder as they amble down the lane.

Friends have assembled for my birthday celebrations. As I drag the closest one from her breakfast, I can scream only disconnected words into her startled face: runaway dogs, must follow, your car." Then I am leaning out the window, pounding on the side of the car, moaning and crying, "My dogs, my dogs." I can't stop myself.

Years ago, I gave a speech at a UNITE gathering for bereaved families. I remember telling them that if we lived in another time and culture, we would be on our knees, pounding the ground, publicly wailing in our grief.

I could imagine that because I could feel that grief. But I had never publicly keened, never expressed that loud, rude, crazy-looking grief for Zachary. Partly because he was already dead when I found out. There was nothing I could do, and that helplessness stunned me into submission.

But it was also true that in those days, I was more restrained by how others were feeling and what they thought. I wanted to be credible in my grief. Not tiresome or hysterical. As if there were a more respectable way to do grief. By being strong, I would be doing right by my son. None of this was conscious at the time. I was certainly in terrible pain, but that habit of being agreeable, being a good soldier, went so deep that I didn't really have a choice.

Not so on the day the greyhounds bolt. It doesn't matter who sees me or what they think of me. I jump in and out of the car. I call for help to passing motorists, screech at anyone who gets in our way. I feel no need to be polite. As I whimper and run through the neighborhood, terrified my greyhounds will become traffic fatalities and I'll never see them alive again, I know I am out of control. And it seems appropriate. As I wail for them, I'm feeling free enough to keen for Zachary in those first awful moments when they told me he was dead.

The greyhounds are fine. I find Strider, call him, and he gallops into my arms. When he and I reach home, Lilith is crossing the lawn to the front door. Both return tired and expecting treats.

# 30

# Photographs

June 2009

The graphic artist at my camera shop specializes in photo restoration. I hand her the Polaroids taken of Zachary at birth. For many years, I've kept them safely tucked away.

These photos had been a complete surprise to me. I didn't know the delivery nurses routinely took pictures of stillborn infants, offered them to the parents, and if the parents didn't want them, kept the photos on file indefinitely. Sometimes, years later, parents would call hoping that the pictures were still available.

The graphic artist looks at the images. "Is the baby...?" She hesitates to finish the question. I shake my head no. "Oh," she says slowly and softly. She scans the photos and we agree that she'll clean up the mottling on his face and correct the uneven lighting.

The first time I saw Zachary, he was curvy shades of gray on a sonogram, a bare bones version of himself, lounging in my uterus while his parts assemble.

My next opportunity was at delivery. Twelve hours of labor are winding down. Lights have dimmed in the birthing suite. A voice from the cluster of professionals at the foot of the table announces, "I see his bum." Then, a question.

"Do you want to watch the delivery in the overhead mirror?"

"No," I say. I am afraid to see him dead.

In a while, another question. "Do you want to hold him?"

"I don't know."

Minutes later, instinct routes fear, and I do know. "Yes. Bring him to me."

After several weeks, finally, the camera shop calls. The photos are ready. I open the envelope and it is like meeting him again. My boy cleans up nicely. He looks more peaceful now.

I keep my favorite photo framed in my bedroom. The picture is different from the sketched portrait I've looked at all these years. More personal and real. The sketch is an idea of my boy. These photos bring him closer.

I don't feel sad when I look at him. Well, maybe sometimes. Mostly, I feel complete.

# 31

# Do You Have Children?

February 2010

For parents who have lost a baby, this isn't a simple question, especially at the beginning.

In the years since Zachary's death, I've tried on many answers to the question. The problem is that there are so many variables: who asks the question, how well do I know the person, is the setting personal or professional, how am I feeling at the time.

It's complicated.

"Do you have children?"

"No. I don't"

During the early grief, I just said no. Unless the question came from a close friend, I wasn't ready to share my feelings or tell our story. But I was denying him. I could feel myself shrink and fade and rage every time I said I didn't have children.

"Do you have children?"

"*Do I have children!?*"

There's something so piercingly direct about the question as it's phrased. It feels like a test, and I am going to fail. Do you *have*? Do you *have* the answer? Do you *have* proper identification? Do you *have* the secret word? Do *you have* what it takes? Do you *have* what just about everybody else *has*?

"Do you have children?"

"Yes, I do."

I walk through my forties and fifties learning how to handle these conversations. In the seconds between question and answer, I feel the chasm opening under us. The questioner doesn't know that we're about to fall into a different conversation than he or she had expected. A conversation that will connect us in an intimate way.

"Do you have children?"

"I did."

It's like I've thrown a bomb into the room. This is no longer a leisurely, getting to know you chat. I've brought in the darkness. The asker backs up, gasps, squints to see me more clearly, wonders what to say next. I feel exposed, embarrassed that I've caused shock and stirred sympathy.

"Do you have children?"

"I had a son, but he died."

How do I answer in a way that tells my story and his? How do I give my child his due in the sixty seconds that I have? Do I show photographs? Do I tell the story of my pregnancy? What is appropriate? I feed them information to get us over the awkwardness: "I'd taken two weeks off before my scheduled Cesarean. I spent the day looking at day care centers and interviewing a pediatrician. That evening, after supper, I noticed there was no movement."

"Do you have children?"

"I had a son, Zachary, but he died two weeks before his due date. It was terrible, but I'm fine now. It's always good to talk about him."

I worry less about the other person and about my own feelings. And I can say his name with pride. The conversation is about him.

"Do you have children?"

"I had a son, Zachary, but he died two weeks before his due date. It was terrible. It's always good to talk about him. He changed my life."

I've found an answer that is simple and complete.

# 32

# Flashback

November 2012

I've only returned to the cemetery once since the funeral, and I have not put a marker on Zachary's grave. But I do want to recognize his having been. I want his name to be somewhere people will see it. Perhaps then it will pass through someone's mind just for the music and goodness of it.

When a senior center in my community is fundraising, I contribute a paving stone that will carry his name: Zachary David Mellon. It isn't a permanent forever thing, but it will last at least as long as I am around.

I teach a memoir class at the senior center. As I'm leaving the building one Monday in November, close to Zachary's 24th anniversary, I stop on the patio to see if the pavers have been installed. They are. At first I can't find his. Have they forgotten us? Then I see it. A rectangular, grey block, very like a grave marker, inscribed "Zachary David Mellon."

A wave of horror crashes over me.

*So, it is true. There was a boy with that name. I do have a son who died.*

I want to run away, but I can't move. It's hard to breathe, as if someone were holding me underwater. My heart is pounding.

*My son is dead. And I've put his name here for everyone to see. What was I thinking? Why have I drawn attention to myself?*

I am back in the nightmare. Grey, anxious days. Shock, disappointment, and terror. The shame of failing at something everyone can do. The way life stops, not only his, but mine, too. The terrible bending it all requires of me.

I stay on the patio until I can breathe again. His name on the stone has dissolved time and place, and has triggered the raw emotional memory I carry in my bones. This isn't the wistful reminiscence I visit when I think of Zachary. This is the original footage. Standing by his stone, I am re-experiencing the trauma of his death with every part of me.

Even after I leave, it takes a while to separate that November twenty-six years ago from this experience with his name on the stone. PTSD doesn't happen only in war zones.

# 33

# A Father's Grief

August 2013

Matt sits on my office sofa with his arm draped around his wife, Barbara. They're an attractive couple in their early thirties, and coming to see a psychologist had not been part of their plan for the month of August. They share a glassy, panicky look as they try to tell the story of their daughter, Sarah, who was stillborn two weeks ago. The pitch of sadness in my office is stunning. Grief times two.

They take turns speaking. It had been a difficult pregnancy: several close calls with pre-term labor, bedrest, daily fear that they would lose the baby. There'd previously been three miscarriages, and they had embarked on this pregnancy as their one last try. With the due date approaching, they'd begun to feel hopeful. Maybe this time.

As Barbara weeps, Matt blinks hard, rubs her shoulder with one hand, and swipes away his own tears with the other. He had made all the hard phone calls after the delivery, arranged the funeral and acted as the go-between in all dealings with the outside world. Barbra's sadness terrifies him, he says. She is usually so strong. When he tries to talk about losing Sarah, his grief chokes him into silence. Barbara says she is worried about him. When will it be his turn to grieve and be taken care of, she wonders. Matt reassures her that he is grieving in his own way.

We talk about how idiosyncratically partners grieve, and look at ways they can bridge their differences to support each other. It's clear that Matt's role as protector gives him solace, and I suggest to them both that they may come to a point when their roles will change.

Several weeks pass and Matt calls and asks if he can come in by himself. He's changed. The rigid, frightened expression is gone from his face. He looks younger and more relaxed, and sadder.

He explains that returning to work has been more difficult than he expected. Concentrating on numbers and dealing with his super-visees exhaust him. People have been especially considerate and that makes him feel awkward, embarrassed. Barbara told him she feels he is drifting away from her. When she asked him to come in and try to talk, he agreed.

And then there was the incident on the golf course. Matt had made time for a game with friends. He'd always played a good game and hoped golf would relax him as it usually had. By the eighth hole, he'd hooked the ball into a tree once and popped it three times. He couldn't find his rhythm. Nothing worked. Everything he tried failed. His frustration erupted, and he found himself beating the ground with his golf club until it was bent and useless.

"I've never been angry like that. I completely lost it. I felt crazy," he says. "Just telling you about it makes me mad. That last popped ball.... My whole life feels like I'm not going anywhere. We've done everything right and we're not getting anywhere. I couldn't keep my own baby safe. I couldn't protect Barbara from all this."

Since the incident, he explains that he's been able to talk a little about the baby with Barbara. He has been able to cry with her. "I wanted to be a good father. I feel useless."

"And angry?" I ask.

"Yes," he says. "Angrier than you can imagine."

We talk about ways Matt can feel his anger without letting it take over. I assure him that he is not crazy. Far from it. He's grieving his child.

# 34

## New Ways of Seeing

March 2014

Over the years, I've had five greyhounds euthanized. They fade away with a soft exhale, and there is that inscrutable stillness. Like a cosmic question just when you need an answer.

At thirteen and a half, Lilith has lived the longest of them all. We've been together for ten years when a cancer-related fracture takes us unexpectedly to the emergency vet. There is nothing to be done but deliver her from the pain.

I never see the departure at these euthanasias. I've always wished I could.

After the vet completes the procedure and leaves us, I sit with her for a while. Then, as I walk to the door, I realize she is still hovering, in a bewildered way, in that bare, green room. I stop. I breath, soften into my impression of her unsettledness.

Part of my brain wonders at what I'm doing. The other part stays with the sensation until that sense of confusion passes. In a few minutes, my body loosens into a more relaxed state. The room feels empty. She is gone. I go home.

To feel presence shift into absence of presence, and to admit that I feel it, are new experiences for me. Zachary's birth and death have made me more sensitive and forced me beyond my usual world of logic and conventionality into the broadened world of intuition and instinct. I'm learning to trust other ways of knowing.

# 35

# Finding Zachary

November 2015

This morning, as I passed Zachary's portrait on the stairway, I smiled, touched the glass, and felt the warmth of our connection. It was spontaneous and deeply satisfying.

I'd been thinking about this book which I now consider our book, our story. Writing *Still Life* has helped me realize how deeply related we are. I can feel now how he has been there all along, changing the shape of my life as surely as he would have altered it in other ways, had he lived.

Zachary's brief life and death compelled me to figure out what was essential to my being and to move toward it in almost every aspect of my life. Spending time with our story has made me more mindful of the changes he fostered in me, changes that now enable me to feel him enlivened in my heart.

I am conscious of his presence, not as a baby now, but as a fellow soul, a guide, and companion. I'm grateful to have him back, my own timeless, ageless bit of starlight that for nine months was a doted-upon human boy.

I imagine that his being is large, and bright, and full of laughter. He doesn't feel like a stranger any more.

# Suggested Reading

Ilse, Sherokee. *Empty Arms. Coping with Miscarriage, Stillbirth and Infant Death.* Maple Plain: Wintergreen Press, Inc., 1982.

Kohn, Ingrid and Moffitt, Perry-Lynn. *A Silent Sorrow. Pregnancy Loss: Guidance and Support for You and Your Family.* New York: Routledge, 2000.

Nelson, Tim. *A Guide for Fathers: When A Baby Dies.* St Paul: 2004.

Wolfelt, PhD, Alan. *Healing a Grandparent's Grieving Heart. 100 Practical Ideas After Your Grandchild Dies.* Fort Collins: Companion Press, 2014.

Klass, Dennis, Silverman, Phyllis R, Nickman, Steven L, eds. *Continuing Bonds. New Understandings of Grief.* Washington, DC: Taylor and Francis: 1996.

Finkbeiner, Ann K. *After The Death of a Child. Living with Loss Through the Years.* Baltimore: John Hopkins University Press, 1998.

# Readers Guide

(Please note that this guide is not meant to replace grief counseling.)

These questions can be used in support group meetings, between partners, among families, friends or in personal reflection. They are designed to facilitate conversations and remembrances that, decades after a stillbirth or miscarriage, rarely, if ever, happen. Spending time with this history confirms and honors the reality of a stillborn's life and death, increases consciousness of your on-going bond, and refreshes your understanding of how this child has influenced your life. These conversations and reflections offer a rare chance to have this child's name spoken and heard.

1. How long ago was your stillbirth?

2. What was the pregnancy like? What are the details you remember about your child's in-vitro life?

3. Where were you and your partner at that point in your lives? Was this a planned child or a surprise?

4. Were there other children or was this your first pregnancy?

5. How did you learn there was a problem?

6. What do you remember about the delivery?

7. Did you see your baby? If so, describe him or her.

8. What did you name the child? How did you choose that name?

9. Do you know why your baby died?

10. Did you have a funeral or a memorial service? What do you remember about it?

11. Tell about the first few weeks after the loss. What or who helped you the most during that time?

12. How did you grieve? How did your partner grieve? If there were other children, how did they grieve?

13. What stands out when you think about that first year? How did you cope?

14. When do you remember beginning to feel better? Can you describe the new normal?

15. Did you have subsequent pregnancies? Describe those experiences.

16. What has been your experience of anniversaries?

17. Do you feel a connection with this child? Can you describe it? How do you nurture it?

18. Have there been moments of feeling your child's presence. If so, can you describe the experience?

19. What do you believe about life after death? How has your loss affected that belief?

20. Does your child's name come up in conversation these days?

21. Do you dream about your child? If so, can you share one of the dreams?

22. How has this child's life and death influenced who you have become spiritually, emotionally, and as a parent and partner? Have you made changes in your personal life or career that you can trace back to this experience?

23. Do you have pictures of your child in the house?

24. What makes you think of your child? Are there people or places or situations that particularly bring him or her to mind?

25. Do you remember your child in a formal way regularly? By a ritual or some other personal gesture?

www.ingramcontent.com/pod-product-compliance
Lightning Source LLC
Chambersburg PA
CBHW031147090426
42738CB00008B/1250